THE GIFT

A Sound Mind for Life

How to increase mental focus, improve memory, and prevent or delay Alzheimer's

Suka Chapel-Horst, RN, PhD, QMHP, CPLT

THE GIFT
A Sound Mind for Life

Author: Suka Chapel-Horst, RN, PhD, QMHP, CPLT

Published by:
Brainworks Publishing
638 Spartanburg Highway, Suite #70-175
Hendersonville, NC 28792

www.IMRIWellness.org
www.AriseAlcoholRecovery.com

Permission granted to copy or reproduce any portion of this transcript.

ISBN-13 978-1494704483
ISBN-10 149470448X

Suka Chapel-Horst

The Gift – A Sound Mind for Life

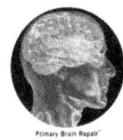

PRIMARY BRAIN REPAIR

Primary Brain Repair focuses on providing the brain, body, and spirit with the basic requirements for health and wellbeing. It's the first line response to all illnesses and disorders. It involves the use of natural micronutrients, nutrition therapy, exercise, and stress relief.

Optimal health can be achieved by most people by following these guidelines. For individuals who need more intensive treatment, these basic health steps will be the foundation that allows advanced treatment to be effective. When primary brain repair is not addressed, medications and counseling have little long-term effect.

Using simple, but effective, recovery tools, *Primary Brain Repair* will improve the health of everyone who applies it. How can that be? Simply, because we go back to the basics of how the brain and body are designed to work. The answer is in nature, and the method is natural.

At Integrative Memory Research Institute our mission and passion is to educate the public and healthcare professionals about the most advanced methods for obtaining optimal health, naturally. Based on the latest neuroscience and biochemical research, along with years of experience, Dr. Suka offers leading-edge knowledge and how-to information to those who are seeking real recovery versus symptom relief.

We are passionate about helping you. That's why we've created self-help books and DVDs to guide you through the process.

www.IMRIWellness.org
417-380-3254

Integrative Memory Research Institute (IMRI) is a non-profit 501c3 organization whose mission is to research, develop, and provide educational programs and healing modalities leading to optimal health.

The Gift – A Sound Mind for Life

INTRODUCTION

We are seeing an enormous increase in the numbers of people diagnosed with dementia and Alzheimer's in the U.S. By 2030 it is expected that 10.8 million Americans will have this diagnosis. Many more will be, and already are, recognizing a decrease in mental acuity and in memory recall, even at much younger ages.

There are preventable reasons for this increase. We can reverse the trend if we change the way our present American culture is headed. Individually, we can make changes in our daily life that will prevent memory loss and dementia, and prevent or delay end stage Alzheimer's.

This Bottom Line Book offers steps one can take to create a sound mind for life. It is truly a gift we can give ourselves.

"Dr. Suka" Chapel-Horst
December 2013
Hendersonville, North Carolina

ABOUT THE AUTHOR

Both of my parents had some dementia at the end of their lives, but not in a serious way. As a nurse working in a nursing home, I was drawn to the old people lined up in rocking chairs in the hallway where they could see the activity at the nurse's station. While they were unable to communicate, it was hoped that the activity would stimulate them in some way. They were waiting for the final call, and for some, the wait was a long time in coming.

Dementia and Alzheimer's present a terrible burden upon the family of the diagnosed person. Caregivers of Alzheimer's patients are six times more likely than the normal population to develop Alzheimer's due to experiencing high levels of chronic stress.

I have watched one of my dear friends slip away over the years. Now, seven years later, she is still with us in the physical but her Spirit has long ago moved into a dimension of peace, I believe. Only her friends and family remain to shoulder the awareness of loss. My husband's father was also a victim of this disorder. It's all too common.

To think that a president of this country could not remember what he had achieved in his lifetime is difficult to comprehend. Dementia and Alzheimer's were not common when I was growing up. Why is it so common now? The answer is not hidden. It's plain before our eyes. That is a good thing. It means we can do something to stop this runaway disorder.

In my forty-plus years of experience as a Registered Nurse and as an ordained inter-faith minister, I've been fortunate to have been introduced to many alternative resources for recovery, and to many healers, researchers, scientists, and leading-edge thinkers. I've brought some of those resources to this presentation. May they be helpful and healing for you, and for your loved ones. *Dr. Suka*

DEDICATION

This Bottom Line Book is dedicated to the 5.4 million Americans who have Alzheimer's. That number is predicted to double by 2030.

The Gift – A Sound Mind for Life

THE GIFT
A Sound Mind for Life

I will begin this little book with a set of questions for an adult of any age. You can add up your "yes" answers as you go through it.

ARE YOU EXPERIENCING COGNITIVE DECLINE?

1. From time to time I forget what day of the week it is.
2. Sometimes, when I'm looking for something, I forget what it is that I'm looking for.
3. My friends and family seem to think I'm more forgetful now than I used to be.
4. Sometimes I forget the names of my friends.
5. It's hard for me to add two-digit numbers without writing them down.
6. I frequently miss appointments because I forget them.
7. I rarely feel energetic.
8. Small problems upset me more than they once did.
9. It's hard for me to concentrate for even an hour.
10. I often misplace my keys, and when I find them, I often can't remember putting them there.
11. I frequently repeat myself.
12. Sometimes I get lost, even when I'm driving somewhere I've been before.
13. I often forget the point I'm trying to make.
14. To feel mentally sharp, I depend upon caffeine.
15. It takes longer for me to learn things than it used to.

Nine or more "yes" answers may be a sign of age-associated memory impairment.

OUR BRAIN

Let's begin with some information about our brain. The outer layer in the front of the brain is the called the neocortex. It's where we think, analyze, intuit, foresee consequences of our actions, and where we learn socially appropriate behavior. Its language is words and numbers. In this area of the brain we have conscious awareness of our emotions and senses and it's the area where we can manage our emotions (if we choose to do so).

The temporal lobe lies on each side of the brain. It's responsible for most memory, hearing, and language. Memory is also stored in every cell in the body, in the DNA.

Within the center of the brain is the limbic system, a primitive brain consisting of the amygdala, hippocampus, hypothalamus, thalamus, and pituitary gland.

The limbic system is the first responder. It's completely instinctual and survival oriented. Its language is the five senses: seeing, hearing, feeling, tasting, and smelling. This is the area that processes memories.

The limbic system is the seat of all emotions, mad, glad, sad, and scared.

A biochemically healthy neocortex can manage emotions, reactions, memory and memory recall but a biochemically compromised brain will be at the mercy of emotions and fight or flight (survival) reactions. This is when memory and memory recall will be jeopardized.

The hippocampus, in the limbic system in the center of the brain, is the brain's memory center. It stores some short-term and a few long-term memories. It ships most long-term memories to the temporal lobe. It stores dry unemotional facts and is the first part of brain to be damaged in Alzheimer's.

The amygdala, in the limbic system, is the main processing area for emotional memories. It helps the hippocampus sort and store memories, especially ones with emotion. It evaluates the emotional impact thoughts carry. The more emotion that is connected with thought, the more likely the memories will be put into long-term storage. Panic, however, can cause amnesia.

The limbic system is linked to the endocrine system which includes eight glands, all producers of hormones. The liver and kidneys also secrete hormones directly into the bloodstream affecting memory.

STRESS EROSION

We live in an age of super stress. Our present population is being decimated by stress and its biochemical ramifications. Today there are more neurological stressors than in the past. Physical stress has largely been replaced by mental and emotional stress but our bodies were not designed for high amounts of emotional stress.

We live in a time of information overload. The average American see's 16,000 advertisements, logos and labels, daily. Add in news messages, radio programs, Muzak, job-related information, movies, books, magazines, and more.

We are victims of technology-induced exhaustion from phones, faxes, computers, TVs, voice mail, email, text messages, portable stereos, car radios, and noise. Plus honking horns, traffic jams, road rage, flashing lights, irritable clerks, put on holds, and loud rap music.

We have to be Supermen and Superwomen to handle Super-Stress due to negative people, job stressors, family discord, multi-tasking, downsizing, competition, economy, health care costs, and government insanity and instability.

So, let's consider the stress response and stress degeneration. The sign on the back of a big truck that's crowding the highway says,

"How's my driving"
TOO SLOW?
Am I impossible
TO OVERTAKE?
Making you later than ever?
FANTASTIC!
Have a nice day.

STRESS AGES,
SICKENS, AND KILLS

According to the CDC and Dr. Bruce Lipton, cellular biologist, stress is responsible for 80-95% of all illness, disease, premature aging, and mental misery.

THE KEY TO A SOUND MIND AND BODY IS STRESS RELIEF

When we are stressed, for any reason, adrenaline is released from the adrenal glands. It's a fight or flight hormone that raises the heart rate, increases blood supply to muscles, increases blood sugar for more energy, and increases blood flow to the brain activating cognitive function and memory recording. Adrenaline prepares the body to respond quickly.

When we're driving and suddenly hear brakes squealing and horns honking, we're able to apply the brakes or swerve almost without thinking because of the adrenaline rush.

At the same time cortisol is released from the adrenal glands. Cortisol is the primary stress responder. While adrenaline is short term, lasting only minutes in the system, cortisol stays in the system much longer, up to hours.

Cortisol is the primary stress responder. It releases blood sugar (glucose) into the blood stream and enhances the brain's use of glucose but it also curbs nonessential activities such as digestion, the reproductive system and growth processes. It also alters immune system function.

Cortisol is not harmful in moderate amounts. However, when it's produced in excess, day after day, as a result of chronic, unrelenting stress, cortisol is so toxic to the brain that it, not only kills and injures brain cells by the billions, but it destroys the biochemical integrity of the brain.

CHRONIC CORTISOL DESTROYS THE BRAIN AND KILLS MEMORIES

Cortisol bathes the hippocampus and other parts of the brain with a highly destructive "toxic bath." Chronic exposure of the brain to toxic levels of cortisol is a primary cause of brain degeneration during the aging process. Even without the toxic effects of cortisol, the hippocampus declines 1% to 2% every year so it's easy to see why chronic exposure to cortisol can be so devastating for the quality of one's life.

Cortisol toxicity is one of the primary causes of Alzheimer's disease. One of eight adults has dementia or Alzheimer's and one of three seniors die with dementia or Alzheimer's. (Other causes appear to be genetic, environmental, metabolic and decreased blood flow to the brain.)

So, how intelligent is our body? Science now has a "new biology" called **EPIGENETICS**, stemming from a combination of biochemistry and quantum physics. It means "control *above* genetics". We used to think that our DNA controlled a large, if not most, of our cellular behavior. Now we know that it only controls a small part of behavior because all cells have an intelligence that responds to the environment.

We can modify genetic behavior without changing genetic blueprints and these modifications can be passed on to future generations. How powerful is that?

For example, DNA is responsible for only 5% of cancers and only 2% of disorders are due to single genes.

The shared physical *environment* and shared *beliefs* of family members are what predispose us to a disease, or outcome. And, we have the ability

17

to change that outcome by changing our physical, mental, and emotional environment. This is a HUGE change in the way we understand the effects of DNA.

We now know that just because people have the gene for Alzheimer's, it doesn't mean they will *get* Alzheimer's. Prevention is possible. 80% of the body doesn't age and can be modified.

Each one of us is the master of 50 trillion cells that have an intelligence that responds to our environment including:
- what we **ingest** - food and drugs
- our **physical** environment - air, viruses, bacteria, molds, toxins, chemicals and
- our **thoughts** - beliefs, assumptions, prejudices, labels, and judgments

All of this means we are much more in control of our fate then we previously thought.

There are approximately 100 billion neurons, or brain cells. They are not connected to each other, being independent entities.

Chemicals called neurotransmitters carry messages (electromagnetic energy) from one neuron to another. These neurotransmitters are made from proteins and all proteins are made up of amino acids.

We're going to look at six neurotransmitters that affect mental focus, concentration, and memory. They are:
- Acetylcholine - "Superstar" Neurotransmitter
- Norepinephrine – "Bright" Neurotransmitter
- Dopamine - "Energizer Bunny" Neurotransmitter
- Serotonin - "Sunshine" Neurotransmitter
- GABA – "Chill Out" Neurotransmitter
- Endorphins – "Love Bug" Neurotransmitters

ACETYLCHOLINE, the "Superstar" neurotransmitter, is the most abundant neurotransmitter in the brain. It's highly concentrated in the hippocampus. It triggers muscle action and concentration.

Symptoms of an Acetylcholine <u>deficiency</u> are:
- Difficulty remembering names and faces, birthdays and numbers
- Difficulty remembering lists, directions or instructions
- Forgetting common facts
- Trouble understanding spoken or written language
- Forget where put things (e.g. keys)
- Make simple mistakes
- Slowed and/or confused thinking
- Difficulty finding right words before speaking
- Disorientation
- Social withdrawal
- Feel despair, lack joy and passion
- Decreased creativity and imagination

The nutrient "Choline" is the primary ingredient of Lecithin.

NOREPINEPHRINE is the "Bright" neurotransmitter (also a hormone). It excites us and elevates our mood. It carries memories from short-term to long-term storage. It helps regulate the sex drive and stimulates the metabolic rate. (Exercise and diet pills elevate norepinephrine, decreasing the appetite.)

Symptoms of a Norepinephrine <u>excess</u> are:
- Memory prevention
- Interferes with rational thought and decision making
- Feeling overwhelmed, frazzled, stressed
- Insomnia
- Decreased sex drive

Nutrients: L-Tyrosine, L-Phenylalanine, Vitamin C, B3, B6, copper

DOPAMINE, the "Energizer Bunny" Neurotransmitter creates:
- Concentration
- Clear thinking
- Memory retrieval
- Feel pleasure
- Energized
- Enthusiastic
- Motivated
- Stimulating
- Stimulates sex drive
- Controls physical movement

Symptoms of a Dopamine <u>deficiency</u> are:
- Difficulty concentrating
- Slowed thinking
- Easily mentally and physically fatigued
- Reduced ability to feel pleasure
- Flat, bored, apathetic and low enthusiasm
- Depressed
- Low drive and motivation
- Procrastination
- Low energy
- Crave caffeine/nicotine/sodas
- Shy/introverted
- Low libido or impotence
- Sleep too much
- Restless leg syndrome
- Trouble getting out of bed
- Put on weight easily

Nutrients: L-Tyrosine, L-Phenyalanine, Co-factors

SEROTONIN is the "Sunshine" Neurotransmitter that helps us to:
- Feel good
- Elevate mood
- Initiate sleep
- Improve dream recall
- Improve appetite
- Decrease emotional pain
- Patience
- Flexibility

Symptoms of a Serotonin <u>deficiency</u> are:
- Inability to concentrate
- Depression
- Anxiety
- Irritability
- Impatience
- Impulsiveness
- Weight gain or unexplained weight loss
- Slow growth in children
- Overeating and/or carbohydrate cravings
- Poor dream recall
- Insomnia

Nutrients: L-Tryptophan, 5-HTP, Co-factors

GABA is the *"Chill Out"* Neurotransmitter that:
- Reduces anxiety (High anxiety levels increase risk of strokes.)
- Eliminates panic
- Emotional relaxation
- Improves sleeping
- Feel good
- Assists Serotonin

Symptoms of a GABA <u>Deficiency</u> are:

- Difficulty relaxing
- Easily stressed or overwhelmed
- Overworked or pressured
- Body uptight or stiff
- Sometimes feel weak or shaky
- Use sugar, alcohol, other drugs to relax
- Increased stress if skip a meal
- Bothered by loud noises, lights, too much activity

Nutrients: Inositol, L-Glutamine, GABA, Co-factors

ENDORPHINS are the "Love Bug" neurotransmitters that:

- Reduce emotional pain
- Reduce physical pain
- Decrease stress and frustration
- Feel comfortable
- Energize
- Elevate focus and concentration

Symptoms on an Endorphin <u>deficiency</u> are:

- Discomfort
- Persistent emotional pain
- Persistent physical pain
- Stress and frustration
- Low interest, focus, concentration

Nutrients: L-Phenylalanine, Co-factors

Posttraumatic Stress Disorder memories are due, in part, to chronically high cortisol levels, excessive Dopamine and Norepinephrine levels, and Endorphin, Serotonin, and GABA deficiencies. (See the Bottom Line Book PTSD in the Resources section of this book for more information.)

Before going further, let me clarify a word that I'll be using as it relates to biochemistry. A "precursor" is a compound that participates in a chemical reaction that produces another compound, for example, hydrogen and oxygen molecules combine to form water.

Some Amino Acid precursors are:
- Lecithin leads to Acetylcholine.
- L-Phenyalanine leads to L-Tyrosine which leads to both L-DOPA and Dopamine which leads to Norepinephrine.
- L-Tryptophan leads to 5HTP which leads to Serotonin.
- Inositol leads to L-Glutamine which leads to the amino acid GABA which leads to the neurotransmitter GABA.
- Phenyalanine leads to the Endorphins.

Examples of chemical imbalances are:

Low Dopamine leads to depression and AD(H)D. Excessive Norepinephrine leads to paranoia and hallucinations. High copper levels are involved with schizophrenia, bipolar disorder, and post-partum depression.

Nootropics is a name for "smart drugs". They enhance cognition and memory with very few side effects. Piracetam, useful in early stage Alzheimer's, is an example of a former prescription drug that is now available over-the-counter.

It's normal for hormone and neurotransmitter production to decrease with age. To achieve physical and brain longevity, it's important to maintain healthy levels of these neurotransmitters.

THE KEYS TO A SOUND MIND FOR LIFE
- Manage Cortisol (the aging hormone) levels by reducing stress.
- Maintain biochemical balance.

Sound Mind Tool Kit
- Neuro-nutrients
- Healthy nutrition
- Physical exercise
- Deep breathing
- Mental exercise
- Meditation and/or mantra
- Belief management
- Visualization

Benefits
- Improve memory
- Sharpen concentration and focus
- Increase learning ability
- Expand problem-solving creativity
- Feel more cheerful and buoyant
- Stabilize endocrine function
- Stop tiring in mid-afternoon
- Increase energy
- Prevent or delay Alzheimer's

Our goal is to age with grace and a sound mind.

THE MAGIC OF AMINOS

The workbook *"Why Do I Feel This Way?" – Natural Healing for Optimal Health and Relief from Moods and Depression* contains a Mood Meter for neurotransmitter testing to find out what, if any, neurotransmitters one may be deficient in. The book also includes amino acid protocols with "what, when, and how" instructions (See page 48 in Resources).

Please don't go out and purchase amino acids without reading the precautions listed in this book. If a person has certain disorders, or is on certain medications, some amino acids should not be taken, or should be taken with care.

Always choose quality over cost when purchasing amino acids and food supplements. Inexpensive aminos and supplements are often made in China. They are cheap because they have no quality control, no supervision, no oversight, and often no amino acids and no herbs in the capsules, regardless of what the written contents state.

Amino acids can't work by themselves. They require partners, or co-factors, to help with their metabolism. Nothing works alone in the body. It takes a village of vitamins, minerals, enzymes, essential fatty acids, trace elements, and herbs to achieve optimal health.

For example, let's look at just the Vitamin B's. When there is a deficiency in these nutrients, multiple symptoms may develop such as:

Emotional Symptoms due to Vitamin B Deficiency:
- Confusion
- Poor concentration
- Poor memory
- Depression
- Insomnia
- Anxiety
- Agitation
- Impulsive
- Anger
- Irritability
- Quarrelsome
- Mood swings
- Panic attacks
- Obsessive-compulsive

Physical Symptoms due to Vitamin B Deficiency
- Hyperactivity
- Headache

- Fatigue
- Insomnia
- Convulsions
- Agitation
- Decreased sex drive
- Tension
- Dizziness
- Gastric ulcers
- High blood pressure
- High cholesterol
- Arteriosclerosis
- Constipation
- Hair loss
- Skin eruptions
- Kidney /Liver impairment
- Extreme nervous exhaustion

Alcohol flushes the amino acids and Vitamin B's out of the body. What does this tell you about why people who are addicted to alcohol have so many emotional and physical symptoms? (For more information refer to the book *How to Quit Drinking for Good and Feel Good* listed in the Resources section of this book.)

(A complete list of neuronutrients for maintaining a sound mind can be found in the Resources part of this book, along with some suggested reference books.)

Americans are the most malnourished people in the world and have the worst diet, according to the latest statistics. Our increasing obesity, diabetes, heart disease, cancer, and Alzheimer rates are a reflection of our current culture.

Farms aren't what they used to be. Crops are devoid of healthy nutrients due to failure to rotate crops, allow land to lay fallow, and the intense use of insecticides, herbicides, and other growth chemicals, not to mention acid rain and poor water quality. The only answer is to "eat organic".

35.7% of Americans are obese, 68% are overweight, and four out of five black women are obese. (Obesity means 20% over normal weight or 30 pounds overweight, depending on sex, height, build, and age.)

Sugar is the #1 destroyer. It's four times more addictive than cocaine. Excess sugar is a drug causing diabetes, cancer, dementia, and Alzheimer's. Food manufacturers attempt to hide the fact that processed food is highly, if not, mostly, sugar. Just look at the growing list of sugar names.

LIST OF JUST SOME SUGAR NAMES

Agave nectar	Demerara Sugar	Golden sugar	Molasses
Barbados Sugar	Dextrin	Golden syrup	Muscovado sugar
Barley malt	Dextran	Granulated sugar	Organic raw sugar
Beet sugar	Dextrose	Grape sugar	Panocha
Blackstrap olasses	Diastatic malt	Grape juice	Powdered sugar
Brown sugar	Diatase	concentrate	Raw sugar
Buttered syrup	D-mannose	HFCS	Refiner's syrup
Cane crystals	Evaporated cane juice	High-Fructose Corn	Rice Syrup
Cane juice crystals	Ethyl maltol	Syrup	Sorbitol
Cane sugar	Florida Chrystals	Honey	Sorghum syrup
Caramel	Free Flowing	Icing sugar	Splenda
Carob syrup	Fructose	Invert sugar	Sucrose
Castor sugar	Fruit juice	Lactose	Sugar
Confectioner'sugar	Fruit juice	Malt syrup	Syrup
Corn syrup	concentrate	Maltodextrin	Table sugar
Corn sweetener	Galactose	Maltose	Treacle
Corn syrup solids	Glucose	Mannitol	Turbinado sugar
Crystalline fructose	Glucose solids	Artificial Maple	Yellow sugar
Date sugar		Syrup	

Sugar abounds in all white foods such as ice cream, pasta, white bread, pizza crust, white rice, white potatoes, and white flour baked goods.

The Standard American Diet, now officially called SAD (and it is) consists of fast foods and junk foods. French Fries, low grade beef hamburgers with processed cheese on white bread, served with a jumbo size cola. Many families live on such non-foods. Chips, candy, cookies, doughnuts, jugs of coffee, and jumbo size bottles of cola are standard fare in many homes.

The solution is to eat three healthy meals every day. Not one or two, but three, and the most important meal is breakfast.

All meals should consist of protein, fats, vegetables, and fruits. We need to eat plenty of healthy protein (source of amino acids, although not nearly enough to restore neurotransmitter levels). Healthy proteins are:

- Nuts
- Beans
- Butter from grass fed cows
- Cheese
- Yogurt
- Non de-natured whey powder
- Fish
- Beef from grass fed cows
- Free range chicken and eggs

And, speaking of eggs, do you remember when we were told not to eat more than two or three eggs a week because of high cholesterol? Another tale told to sell drugs. Before the statin (cholesterol) drugs, a healthy cholesterol level was 130. When the statin drugs were unleashed on Americans, the AMA was lobbied and induced to lower the "healthy" cholesterol level to 100, where it is today, so that these drugs could be promoted. We now have proof that statin drugs increase:

- Memory loss
- Alzheimer's
- Diabetes
- Hormonal imbalances
- Cancer
- Parkinson's
- Stroke
- Depression
- Suicide
- Violent behavior

According to Dr. Mercola, 95% of people should not be taking statin drugs. Statin drugs have not lowered or decreased heart-related disease, as they were advertised to do. The only decrease is in our pocketbooks.

According to neurologists, the cholesterol in eggs is good for the brain. So, enjoy your breakfast. My husband and I eat breakfast for dinner, quite often.

Two Tips:
1. Omega 3 fish oil with DHA can reduce cortisol levels.
2. A high fat / low refined carbohydrate diet reduces chances of dementia by 44% according to the Mayo Clinic. Eat plenty of nuts, butter, chicken with skin and fat, and of course, chicken soup. (Chicken soup is good for the soul, so the book says, and it just might be true.)

In addition, it's very important to avoid GMO (Genetically Modified Organism) foods. They consist of corn, soy, cottonseed, canola oil, sugar beets, Hawaiian papaya, and some zucchini and squash. Soy is especially detrimental, especially to newborn babies and young children. (See *"Why Do I Feel This Way?"* on page 48.)

Allergies, alone, can be responsible for almost all symptoms. Allergies to wheat and dairy are the most common. The manual mentioned above includes both a written test and instructions for food elimination tests for allergies. Simple, costing nothing, these tests may lead to the resolution of many symptoms and disorders.

It's time to cut down on grains. Unless breads and cereals are made from sprouted grains, the following chain-reactions created by grain consumption are shown to increase the risk of:
- Anxiety (raises cortisol levels)
- Diabetes (raises cortisol levels)
- Depression (leads to sugar cravings raising cortisol levels)
- Autism
- Allergies
- Infertility
- Obesity
- Arthritis

- Schizophrenia (100% are allergic to gluten. Once off gluten, some schizophrenics are completely symptom free.)
- Autoimmune diseases
- Various cancers including: Pancreatic, Colon, Stomach and Lymphoma

Water
Drink six to eight glasses of water every day. Our bodies are about 70% water. When the level is too low we can experience stress related symptoms.

Peridontal care during middle age and onward will help to prevent systemic, or whole body, inflammation which leads to both high cholesterol deposits and also to Alzheimer's disease.

Stretching
Stretching isn't about building muscle or losing weight. It's about maintaining a flexible spinal column. The nervous system flows through the spine and when we become stiff and inflexible, the integrity of the spine is compromised, and so is our life. Daily stretching in the morning before other activities can be a life saver, in so many ways.

Tibetan Five Movements
You will look and feel 10-20 years younger if you practice these five movements every day. I've been doing them for eight years and this is indeed true. You can learn about them in the book *Ancient Secret of the Fountain of Youth* by Peter Kelder with a forward by Bernie Siegel, MD.

Avoiding dementia and stopping premature aging doesn't happen just because we want it to. There are steps and practices we need to take to stay young. But, isn't it worth the effort? Indeed, most people come to fully enjoy their healthy practices and wouldn't quit doing them for anything. They feel too wonderful.

Exercise or walking is a major part of keeping the mind and body alive, alert, and healthy. People who do *moderate exercise* are 39% less likely to get mild cognitive impairment. People who exercise just twice a week has been shown to decrease the *risk* of Alzheimer's by 60%. However, I know that many people don't like to exercise. For those who do, fine. For those who don't, forty minutes of brisk walking four days a week will do it. Keeping the heart rate up and breaking a little sweat is a good sign that you're getting a decent workout.

Yoga, Tai Chi, and Qigong are excellent ways of reducing stress. Additional methods help to release toxins and stress from the body. They are excellent adjuncts to emotional energy releasing work.

- Reiki
- Massage
- Reflexology
- Chiropractic
- Acupuncture
- Quantum Touch
- Polarity Therapy
- Therapeutic Touch
- Cranial Sacral Therapy
- Myofascial Trigger Point
- Infra-Red Dry-Heat Saunas

Breathing for stress relief is free and it's the easiest, most natural, and BEST method for reducing stress. Most people are breathing in such a way that they are actually inducing a stress response. Whenever we breathe short, shallow breaths in the top of our lungs and then hold our breath, we're creating stress. This kind of breathing leads to anxiety and eventually to fear.

Instead, take slow, deep, and regular breaths, drawing the air down into the bottom of your lungs, allowing the rib cage to expand. This changes the brain chemistry to allow for relaxation. The manual I've mentioned earlier has seventeen stress-reducing exercises, some of which are about breathing.

ABOUT THE MIND

Mental exercise can keep the brain alert. We know that frequently after retirement, people can become bored, and, without mental stimulation, they rapidly age, losing their mental acuity. To avoid this, stimulate your brain with any exercises that use language, numbers, reasoning, and spatial organization. Video games have been shown to increase cognition. Here are some other ideas.

Reading	Conversing
Writing	Take classes
Drawing	Puzzles
Word games	TV quiz shows
Board games	TV Documentaries
Card games	Sports
Building	Games
Stimulating hobbies	Volunteer

Music, combined with movement, will also increase cognition. Playing a musical instrument, dancing, or just moving with music is helpful. Drumming is another excellent way to maintain mental abilities.

There is no reason to stop learning and productivity after retirement. Retirement may be a change of focus but it's also an opportunity to follow your bliss. Get excited about a new project and give it your all. Instead of planning for "the end", take advantage of all the years you have to make a difference in the world. The planet couldn't exist without all the volunteering people do. Instead of a rocking chair,... you rock.

Mental memory tips can help but they don't increase memory ability. Only rebalancing brain chemistry using the micronutrients and healthy nutrition, along with exercise, and mental stimulation will do that. However, these tips can be used to aid in memory recall.

1. **Multiple associations** – What else is connected to it? Make a grocery list by visualizing items stacked together, such as placing potatoes inside a box of laundry soap, which is placed between

slices of bread, and so on. It's not logical but the image can stick long enough to get through the shopping event.

2. **Attaching emotion** – Sends to long-term memory. Just met a new person and want to remember his name? How does he make you feel? Comfortable, humorous, uneasy? Feel the emotions while repeating his name. Often, we aren't in touch with our emotions and so, we lose the information. Stay in "feel".

3. **Multiple encoding** – Add auditory and visual stimuli. Want to remember a restaurant you just ate at? What were the sounds in the room? Soft or noisy? Was music playing? Were there sounds from the kitchen? Look at the patrons. Are they wearing coats? Are they more young or more old, or both? Do they seem happy, worried, chatty, bored? What were the wait people wearing? Were they attentive? ...and so on.

4. **Chunking** – Group into sevens. Telephone numbers are grouped into sevens for better memory.

5. **Review** – Review three to five times. Repeat or reread the information with concentration.

6. **Conscious forgetting** – Make a list and write it down.

7. **Concentration** – Make an EFFORT to concentrate.

Memory is a skill that can be improved as we age. It isn't necessarily tied to one's IQ. Isn't that good news?

Reduce stress by changing how you think. We cause stress by how we think about something. If we stopped labeling, judging, making assumptions, and jumping to negative conclusions, our stress levels would diminish or disappear.

Over-generalizing by using the words "always, never, and everybody" makes mountains out of molehills. And then there's the "kitchen sink arguments" that begin small and escalate to include "all the dirty dishes in the sink" or every little irritant that lies just below the surface. It all comes pouring out and the repercussions can be overwhelming. Cortisol flows for hours after one of these arguments.

Awfulizing is another way to build stress, especially when situations are considered to be awful, terrible, impossible, or horrendous. It may be an opportunity, a challenge, or offer a new and better direction. For example, "If my beloved dog hadn't been in a terrible accident, I wouldn't have met the veterinarian who I fell in love with and eventually married."

BUBBLE OF PROTECTION

This exercise is covered more fully in the aforementioned self-help manual. Basically, imagine a Plexiglas bubble surrounding you. No one can see it and no one needs to know you have imagined it there.

While standing and imagining this bubble around you, reach out and feel its imaginary surface. Feel above you, and all around the sides. Notice whether it feels warm or cold. Do you hear an imaginary sound as you rub your hands over its surface? Of course, you can see right through it.

This bubble allows all good thoughts, including caring and love to pass through it easily. But negative thoughts can't pass through. So, as you go about your daily life, any negativity that comes toward you will hit your bubble and be thrown back to the sender, where it belongs, anyway. You will be protected. Sound crazy? Well, it works.

It works because of your intention. Doing the imaginary "feel" imprints the image into your kinesthetic memory and makes it "real" to your subconscious mind. Once you have done the preliminary "feel", all you have to do is mentally place yourself into the bubble when you get up in the morning and you'll be protected all day.

Do this daily for a week. Notice the difference. You'll see that it works. Professional ballplayers use this method very successfully to imagine their plays and train their bodies to respond. It hugely improves their actual playing ability.

Note that your negativity will remain inside the bubble with you, which is good. You can notice it and change it. Try it. You'll like it.

MEDITATION and MANTRA

A 2013 Harvard study showed that eight weeks of mindful meditation (focused, mantra, breathing) increased cognitive ability in Alzheimer's patients. There are many forms of meditation. Focusing on one's breathing is an excellent meditation. Hundreds, perhaps thousands, of books and teachers are available to guide one in meditation. No form is better than any other. Meditate in the manner that resonates most with you. But know that meditation is a very powerful and easy way to drop cortisol levels and decrease damage to your brain cells.

Mantras are words or phrases that are repeated over and over to still the mind and create a peaceful feeling. The words can be any that give you a relaxing feeling. A Catholic might repeat, "Holy Mary, Mother of God." Some might prefer saying a name of God, such as Allah, Jehovah, Jesus, or Buddha. Some might like words such as "peace", "love", or "Om". It doesn't matter what the words are as long as they bring comfort and relaxation.

ROOT OF STRESS

The root of stress is unhealthy beliefs about ourselves, our life, or other people that create inappropriate fear and block us from receiving our prosperity.

Our beliefs come from our parents, family members, teachers, religious training, entertainment, books, TV, and personal trauma. In the first seven years of our life, we don't yet have the ability to discriminate. We accept and believe everything we see, hear, and experience.

These beliefs become subconscious but they control our reactions and actions throughout our life, outside of our awareness. When we are stressed, it's because of a belief we have about that situation. Constant stress means we need to consider what the underlying beliefs are that are causing constant stress. Are those beliefs still valuable today or are they holding us back?

Feeling unworthy may be the most common and destructive belief we can have. If we feel unworthy, we may experience lack of abundance, or lack of opportunities, or lack of friendships, or lack of a healthy relationship.

A major belief source comes from our biological mother during gestation. We are one with the mother during these nine months and we're bathed in her emotions even as they are embedded in our own cellular memory.

Just as she received emotional memories from her mother, and onward back through centuries, we all carry these ancestral cellular memories within us. They prod us to act and react in ways that we often don't understand. We say, "Why did I do that?" but there's no obvious answer.

These cellular memories are stored in every cell in our body within the DNA. They aren't *our* memories and we don't want to continue to carry them forward. Why? Because...

Destructive cellular memories and beliefs are stressors that release cortisol, suppress the immune system, and are the source of all illness and disease, including aging and memory loss.

What were the primary memories that were laid down in your life? Were they ... Mad? Glad? Scared? Sad? How are these memories affecting you now?

The conscious mind is only 5% of our being. The unconscious mind is 95% of who we are and when there is conflict between what we **think** we believe and what we **really** believe, the unconscious mind **always** wins!!!!!

We need to release negative beliefs, habits, and thoughts that no longer serve us well. Create new beliefs of possibility, appreciation, gratitude, and an expectation of prosperity in all things good.

The first step is forgiveness. We can't move forward without both self and other forgiveness but that seems so difficult to do. When we understand the concept that we are all one in the cosmic soup, simply being energy, we can have a fresh perspective on forgiveness.

In the book, ZERO LIMITS, Joe Vitale and Ihaleakala Hew Len, MD, a psychiatrist in Hawaii, write about an ancient forgiveness practice from the South Pacific Islands called **Ho'oponopono**. You will want to find out how Dr. Len was able to release all the hardened criminals in a prison psychiatric ward back to the public as reformed individuals due to this simple and powerful forgiveness healing method.

EXCUSES BEGONE and WISHES FULFILLED by Dr. Wayne Dyer are excellent resources for getting rid of destructive and unhealthy beliefs.

THE FOUR AGES OF HEALING
1. Prayer Healing
2. Herbal Medicine
3. Pharmaceutical Medicine
4. Energy Medicine / Energy Psychology

When human civilization was young, healing was accomplished by praying and sacrificing to animal spirits, nature spirits, and to the sun, moon, and stars.

The second age of healing came when shamans, healers, mid-wives, medicine men and women used herbal remedies. That age lasted into the 1800s.

The third age of healing came with the advent of biochemistry and pharmaceuticals. Today, it's the prevailing method of healing.

However, we are already entering into the fourth age of medicine and healing, the age of energy medicine. The first biofeedback machines are rapidly being replaced by much more sophisticated electronic technologies focused on energy waves. Many healing techniques are available where the practitioner manipulates energy with their hands and mind. Transformational psychology, Hakomi, and other systems are focused on removing energy blocks that inhibit health.

It would seem that we are now entering a time when we can bring what has worked from all the ages together. Prayer, herbal remedies, pharmaceuticals, and energy healing. The next few years will find us moving away from some of the questionable pharmaceuticals and incorporating more of the natural building blocks of nature, such as the amino acids and healthy nutrition. We can take advantage of all of these healing methods right now. I'll introduce you to two systems that I recommend to be very helpful.

EMOTIONAL FREEDOM TECHNIQUES

Developed by Gary Craig, this may be the most effective energy technique available today. By tapping on various points on the head and upper chest, energy blocks are permanently released. This technique is being successfully used with veterans who have PTSD. For more information go to www.eftuniverse.com.

INTEGRATIVE MEMORY THERAPY®

See page 47 in the Resources section for information about this powerful resource for discovering the underlying *unconscious* memories that are responsible for many of our moods, behaviors, and physical health issues.

VALIDATION THERAPY
Developed by Naomi Feil

"A method for communicating with very old people who are diagnosed with dementia." Naomi Feil

This therapy, which everyone can learn, will make caring for a person with dementia or Alzheimer's much easier. You will learn how to keep communication open for an extended period of time. If you know a person diagnosed with severe dementia or Alzheimer's, please go to this web site and watch a 15 minute video. This beautiful method is being taught world-wide for people caring for those with Alzheimer's disease. www.vfvalidation.org.

SUMMARY
The brain is an organ that requires neuronutrients, healthy nutrition, stimulation, rest, relaxation, proper medical care, and support.

Remember Brylcreem? "A little dab'l do ya..." In the case of maintaining a sound mind for life, a little dab won't do it. We have to apply many techniques, however, there are many options available for maintaining a youthful mind, and that's good news.

SUPPORT

I hope you will share this information with others. Find those who are eager to improve their lives and are willing to do what it takes to maintain a sound mind for life. Together, we can avoid, or at the least, delay the effects of an aging mind. It's more than worth the effort, wouldn't you agree?

RESOURCES

The Gift – A Sound Mind for Life

A SOUND MIND FOR LIFE SUGGESTED SUPPLEMENTS

MULTIPLE VITAMIN with magnesium, selenium, and zinc

VITAMIN B6   50 MG 3 x DAILY

VITAMIN B12 (Sublingual) 1000 MCG DAILY

VITAMIN B COMPLEX

VITAMIN C 1000 MG 3 X DAILY

VITAMIN D3   5,000 IU UP TO 40,000 IU DAILY

VITAMIN E 400 IU (2000 IU daily improves cognition in Alzheimer's patients)

COENZYME Q10   100 MG DAILY IN AM

OMEGA 3 + DHA 1000 MG 2X DAILY (Increases brain size in elderly)

DHEA 25-50 MG DAILY AFTER LAB TEST

GREEN DRINK (See Renewal Greens below)

INOSITOL POWDER (Sublingual) 1000 MG 1-4 X DAILY

GINKO BILOBA 160 MG DAILY IN DIVIDED DOSES

GINSENG 750 MG DAILY

BACOPA 500 MG DAILY*

LECITHIN 1,000-1,500 MG 2 X DAILY

PHOSPHATIDYL SERINE 100 MG 2 X DAILY

ACETYL L-CARNITINE 250 MG 1-2 X DAILY

*BACOPA - Please consult your healthcare provider before taking this supplement if you are pregnant or breastfeeding. Bacopa may increase the effects of anti-anxiety, anti-epileptics, tranquilizers, barbiturates, benzodiazepines, narcotics and/or other prescription or OTC medications taken for a health condition.

AMINO ACIDS – See the WorkBook *"Why Do I Feel This Way?"* - *Natural Healing for Optimal Health and Relief from Moods and Depression* on page 48.

RECOMMENDED RESOURCES

BRAIN LONGEVITY SUPPLEMENTS
Dr. Dharma   800-651-5650
www.drdharma.com
Memory Caps
Super Rejuvenation Caps
Gold Caps Multi Vitamin/Mineral

TO ORDER HIGH QUALITY SUPPLEMENTS LISTED IN THIS BOOK, CALL ANOVA HEALTH AT 864-408-8320.

Food supplements listed in all of our books can be purchased through Anova Health, also providing WHOLE FOOD supplements. Request a catalog.

Simply call Anova Health and give them the CODE. **Drsuka5** Your order will be shipped the same day, no delays. You will automatically receive a **5% discount and free shipping,** saving you the extra cost of buying supplements of the very best quality. To get these benefits, you must call in your order.

All supplements are of the highest quality available and are suitable for vegetarians. They are free of wheat gluten, soy, milk/dairy, corn, sodium, sugar, starch, artificial coloring, preservatives, and flavoring. I highly recommend the following supplements available through Anova Health.

Amino Acids: All of the amino acids that are listed in my two "how-to" manuals and other books can be ordered through Anova Health. Of course, they can be purchased in many other places, but for the highest quality and purest products, I recommend Anova Health. You may pay a little more, but you will use less and get better results with high quality products.

AvinoCort for managing elevated Cortisol levels caused by chronic stress. Lowering one's cortisol level slows down the aging process and helps to prevent dementia and Alzheimer's. Why use this product? This is a very advanced, stem cell product. Ask the folks at Anova Health for more information if you like. I highly recommend this product for reducing the effects of chronic stress.

Inositol Powder is a normal vitamin B. It is a precursor to GABA, the brain's natural Valium. If you have anxiety, worries, even panic attacks, your inositol level is probably too low. Taking 1000 mg up to four times daily can improve relaxation and reduce anxiety, naturally.

High Potency Hemp Oil with Cannabidiol (CBD): Legal everywhere and has no measurable THC or psycho-active effects. Cannabidiol relieves or cures over 100 symptoms and disorders. Comes as oil and capsules. An excellent balm is also available for topical use. To learn more about the advantages of hemp oil with Cannabidiol versus marijuana with TCH for medicinal support, order the Bottom Line Book *Cannabinoids – The Hundredth Monkey Cure* (see page 54) available on our web site. This product, combined with vitamin D3, may be the closest there is to "magic medicine". Recommended for drug and alcohol detoxing and recovery, as well.

CaliQuil - California Poppy 500 mg Capsules Restores Rest. Prevails over pain. Traditional analgesic and sleep aid. This amazing product really works. Take it before bedtime and see the results. (Does not produce opium, physical dependence, or addiction.)

Acute Pain Relief, a King Bio homeopathic cream, gives excellent relief from joint pain.

Call 864-408-8320 to order these and other products from Anova Health. (If you order on-line, you won't get the discount or free shipping.)

Use the code **drsuka5** to order.

OTHER SUGGESTED RESOURCES FOR QUALITY SUPPLEMENTS
Call and request free catalogs. Order by telephone or on-line.

Life Extension: www.lef.org 1-800-678-8989

Bronson Vitamins: www.bronsonvitamins.com 1-800-235-3200

Cayenne Company: www.cayennecompany.com 1-800-229-3663

For highest quality amino acids call: Dr. Suka at 417-380-3254 or 417-894-8501

ALCOHOL RECOVERY PROGRAMS

ARISE **Alcohol Recovery** offers two Do-It-Yourself, at home, recovery programs. These include both a Self-Managed Program and a Managed Program.

ARISE **Alcohol Recovery** also offers an Out-patient Program for individuals who have been through one or more treatment programs, or have made good attempts at recovery through AA, and have relapsed. The program can also serve as an aftercare program for someone coming out of treatment but who is not yet ready to return home.

All programs are based on biochemical restoration of the brain using micronutrient and nutrition therapy, body work, whole life skills, and Integrative Memory Therapy®.

For more information and testimonials, go to:
www.AriseAlcoholRecovery.com

INTEGRATIVE MEMORY THERAPY®

Present day physical, emotional, and mental pain and suffering are the result of unresolved issues from our past. It can be called Post Traumatic Stress. That "past" can be yesterday, or years ago. The unresolved issues may have occurred during our early formative years or in the womb.

Yes, we recorded the feelings, thoughts, and words mother experienced during the time we were a tiny fetus in her womb. We simply recorded these, and all that we saw, heard, and felt during the first seven years of our life. These experiences became our history and our truths because we didn't yet have a conscious mind to discriminate. The stories created beliefs about ourselves and our ability to live in the world, even though the beliefs may have been wrong or harmful.

Sometimes these memories or "stories" may appear to be past life trauma stories that are seeking resolution. It makes no difference whether the stories are fantasy or real. If the stories coming from our own unconscious mind are left unresolved, they create unhealthy survival patterns and suffering in our present lives. These unhealthy survival patterns can show up as addictions, cancer, arthritis, anorexia, depression, PTSD, AD(H)D, for example. In fact, every illness and every disorder is the result of unresolved prior trauma.

Integrative Memory Therapy® gets to the originating source of present day issues, allowing for healing and transformation. Unlike other medical and alternative modalities, this process resolves the root of the problem. Healing in the present takes place because the underlying cause is no longer present.

Integrative Memory Therapy® is not regression, nor is it hypnosis. Clients are fully conscious at all times. The therapist guides clients to resolve their own source traumas. The result is a transformed life in the present. This therapy must be conducted in person. It cannot be conducted via Skype or telephone.

For more information contact Dr. Suka at 417-890-3254 or go to www.IMRIWellness.org. More information and testimonials are available on the web site.

RECOMMENDED BOOKS, DVDs

WORKBOOK   (180 pages)
"Why Do I Feel This Way?" -
Natural Healing for Optimal Health and Relief from Moods and
Depression
by Suka Chapel-Horst, RN, PhD, QMHP, CPLT

Moods, cravings, chronic depression, aches, pains and other symptoms are caused by treatable and reversible deficiencies in brain chemistry.

If your brain is low in "feel good" chemicals, you may experience moodiness, sadness, anxiety, overeating, insomnia, irritability, anger, lack of focus and concentration, poor memory, loneliness, decreased sex drive, lack of motivation, racing thoughts, suicidal thoughts, and more.

Find out which "feel good" brain chemicals you may be deficient in. Experience the power of amino acids to restore brain chemistry without medications. Discover the foods and basic food supplements that can restore your life to normal. The guidelines are clear, easy to understand and follow. This book may be all you need to achieve optimal health.

Avoid medication side effects, serious dangers, and addictive qualities. The only way to restore optimal health is by deleting poisonous nonfoods and feeding the brain the natural substances it needs to function normally.

The book includes:
- Ten Written Tests to Uncover the Underlying Cause
- Neurotransmitter Testing
- Amino Acid Formulas
- Nutritional Co-Factor Formulas
- Three Nutritional Programs
- Allergy and Candida Repair
- Seventeen Fun and Effective Stress-Reducing Exercises

WORKBOOK (179 pages)
How to Quit Drinking for Good and Feel Good
by Suka Chapel-Horst, RN, PhD, QMHP, CPLT

Live at Home

Keep it Private

Continue Normal Activities

Make it Affordable

Much of what we thought we knew about alcoholism and substance abuse is now obsolete. Neuroscience and biochemistry have found the underlying cause of all addictions and thirty-plus years of experience have given us the recovery method that is getting up to 85% recovery rates.

Shame, blame, and guilt be gone. Anger and hurt can change to healing, compassion and forgiveness when the real cause of addictions is understood. Addictions are not caused by a mental illness, nor are they caused by a lack of will power, a character defect, or a moral weakness.

Sobriety is not recovery. "One day at a time" struggling, white knuckling, dry drunk behaviors, depression, insomnia, anxiety, cravings, and other symptoms lead to relapse. With the new understanding of addictions, these, and other symptoms can be relieved and prevented, naturally, without the side effects and addictive qualities of prescription medications.

This book contains ten written tests to determine one's underlying biochemical imbalances, plus individual neurotransmitter tests, and a step-by-step guide for gaining and maintaining lasting recovery without the symptoms that lead to relapse. Normal brain chemistry is restored with the natural building blocks of amino acids, micronutrients and healthy nutrition. This program uses the most successful method of recovery available anywhere. Motivated and determined individuals can recover once and for all.

Written tests included in this book are:
- Alcohol Screening
- Carbohydrate Addiction
- Hypoglycemia
- Hypothyroid
- Candida
- Allergies
- Pyroluria
- High Histamine
- Low Histamine
- Attention Deficit (Hyperactivity) Disorder
- Neurotransmitter Deficiencies

DVD
Depression Cure
Ten Different Sources / Ten Different Approaches   Get Real Results
Your Guide to Finding and Treating the Real Underlying Cause
PowerPoint Presentation by Suka Chapel-Horst, RN, PhD, QMHP, CPLT

Don't waste time using the wrong approach to recovery. "Dr. Suka" pinpoints the different underlying sources of depression which must be treated uniquely and appropriately in order to fully recover without the use of pharmaceuticals. These inter-related causes require different treatment approaches to achieve permanent cure. Don't waste precious time, money, and hopes. Get to the root source from the start and find out how to recover naturally. DVD comes with a resource list.

BOOK (234 pages)
Take a Leap of Faith
Wellness Simplified
by Suka Chapel-Horst, RN, PhD, QMHP, CPLT

If your emotional, mental, or physical health isn't what you wish it to be, you'll find practical suggestions for regaining or maintaining optimal health in this remarkable book. The topics include:

- Halt Premature Aging Now
- Want More Sunshine in Your Life?
- The Cookie Monster - Hypoglycemia
- Five Simple Steps to Optimal Health
- Enjoy Life More
- Your Body Type: Seven Dwarfs and Superman
- Fear versus Love
- Relief from Depression
- Stretching to Wellness
- Bodyguards Got You Covered?
- Bodyguard Banquet
- What are you Hoarding in your Mental House?
- Prevent Dementia and Alzheimer's
- The Hundredth Monkey Cure – Cannabinoids
- Is There a Cure for Alcoholism?
- Color – The Hidden Persuader
- The Ultimate Healing – Integrative Memory and Past Lives Therapy®
- Take a Leap of Faith
- What I know for Sure
- ...and more

In the most delightful and warm way, Dr. Suka "talks" about the topics closest to our minds and hearts.   This book includes transcripts from 24 of her recent Unity.FM international radio shows. You won't want to put this book down.

BOTTOM LINE BOOKS

BOOK/DVD
Wellness Simplified
How Food affects Moods, Bodies and Behaviors
PowerPoint Presentation by Suka Chapel-Horst, RN, PhD, QMHP, CPLT

Think what you eat doesn't matter? Fast food, junk food, sodas, and pizza are the voices of violence, crime, and suicide, as well as obesity, joint pain, insomnia, anxiety, diabetes, depression, cancer, and *you name it!*

What we eat affects the quality of our lives. Sick and tired of feeling sick and tired? Are children's behaviors getting out of hand? Are school grades going down? It's OK. There's a solution and it's not rocket science.

This little book can change lives for the better, right now. The solution makes sense and it's doable. Say "goodbye" to moods, sickness, and unwanted behaviors. Say "hello" to good health and happiness.

BOOK
Say Goodbye to Moods and Depression
by Suka Chapel-Horst, RN, PhD, QMHP, CPLT

The only way to restore optimal health is by deleting poisonous nonfoods and feeding the brain the natural substances from which it is made.

Babies are made from food, not Prozac. After birth, why do we switch from the natural building blocks of life to synthetic pills? We can achieve optimal health when we remove the underlying brain chemical imbalances which lead to the symptoms of moods and depression including insomnia, anxiety, panic reactions, irritability, weight gain, aches and pains, and more.

The good news is that targeted micronutrients and healthy nutrition, along with other holistic methods of healthcare, can reduce or eliminate moods and depression, naturally.

BOOK
The Real Cause and Solution for Alcohol Addiction
The NEW Alcoholism Story
by Suka Chapel-Horst, RN, PhD, QMHP, CPLT

Alcohol addiction is caused by an inherited and genetically caused imbalance of brain chemistry. It's not caused by a character defect, a moral shortcoming, or by a lack of will power.

Neuroscience and biochemistry have proven, once and for all, that all addictions are biochemically caused. It's time to give up shame, blame, and guilt for a disorder that is biochemically caused.

When dysfunctional brain chemistry is restored to normal, relapse and dry-drunk symptoms are rare. Learn how imbalanced brain chemistry leads to alcoholism and discover the recovery method that has the highest long-term relapse-free recovery rate.

BOOK
Cannabinoids – The Hundredth Monkey Cure
by Suka Chapel-Horst, RN, PhD, QMHP, CPLT

The human body naturally produces cannabis-like chemicals that keep all body systems in balance. This internal cannabinoid system may be the most important health discovery of recent years. THC, CBN, and CBD from the cannabis sativa plant mimic our internal chemicals and work to improve our overall health. Cannabidiol, or CBD, cures or relieves symptoms of over 100 disorders. ...and it's legal everywhere because it doesn't have the psycho-active ingredient, THC.

Want better natural solutions for your health concerns? This DVD shows how to change brain chemistry and improve your life by using Cannabidiol (CBD), amino acids, neuronutrients, nutrition, exercise, and chronic stress reducers. Say goodbye to anxiety, stress, depression, insomnia, pain, physical disorders, and much more.

BOOK
PTSD – Post-Traumatic Stress Disorder
Alternative Resources for Recovery
by Suka Chapel-Horst, RN, PhD, QMHP, CPLT

Medications have long term, harmful side effects, including addiction, and traditional counseling methods are often only partially effective.

There are two underlying causes of PTSD. 1) Biochemical deficiencies, or brain chemistry imbalances, and 2) underlying, UNCONSCIOUS, unresolved trauma which occurred PRIOR to the known trauma-experience that *appears* to be the cause of PTSD. These unconscious memories are called *source trauma.*

Addressing biochemical, nutritional, brain wave state, and bioenergy fields is a necessary component to recovery, including the clearing of destructive cellular memories using the latest science of energy psychology.

Uncovering and resolving hidden source trauma, the underlying cause of PTSD, is accomplished with *Integrative Memory Therapy®.* (See page 39 in this Appendix.)

BOOK
Trick or Treat – What Your Doctor isn't Telling You about Mood Altering Medications
by Suka Chapel-Horst, RN, PhD, QMHP, CPLT

Is your doctor treating you or tricking you? If you are considering taking mood altering medications, are already on them, or want to get off them, you need to know what these medications are really doing to brain chemistry. Be informed in order to make wise decisions. Your emotional and mental life is at stake.

These books and DVDs can be ordered through:
www.IMRIWellness.org
www.AriseAlcoholRecovery.com
Or by calling: 417-380-3254

Suka Chapel-Horst

The Gift – A Sound Mind for Life